I0423220

PROMOTION & CONSERVATION OF HEALTH, STRENGTH & ENERGY

(Original Version, Restored)

by

LIONEL STRONGFORT

Originally published in 1930

PUBLISHED BY O'Faolain Patriot L L C, Copyright 2012

info@physicalculturebooks.com

ISBN-13: 978-1470105945

ISBN-10: 1470105942

Published in the United States of America

To Order More Copies Visit:
PhysicalCultureBooks.com

1

appropriate for the reader's needs or expectations. The publisher expressly disclaims any and all responsibility and/or liabilities that might result from the uninformed or misinformed application of the techniques identified herein as well as for any unsupervised physical fitness training.

Finally, the publisher disclaims any and all liabilities arising from the use of any equipment featured in this book and makes no representations as to the utility, safety, or adequacy of the equipment generally or with respect to any specific purpose.

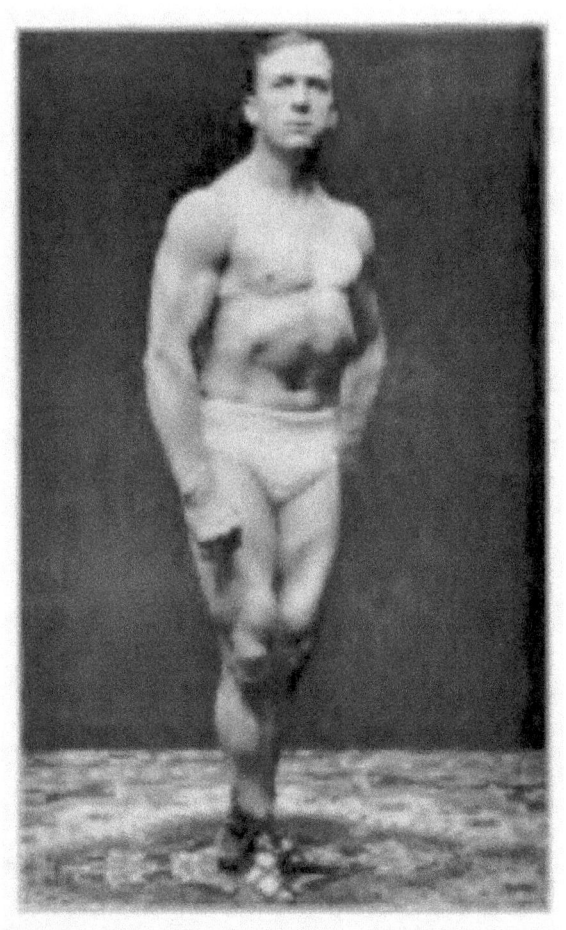

LIONEL STRONGFORT
FOUNDER
The Source of Strongfortism

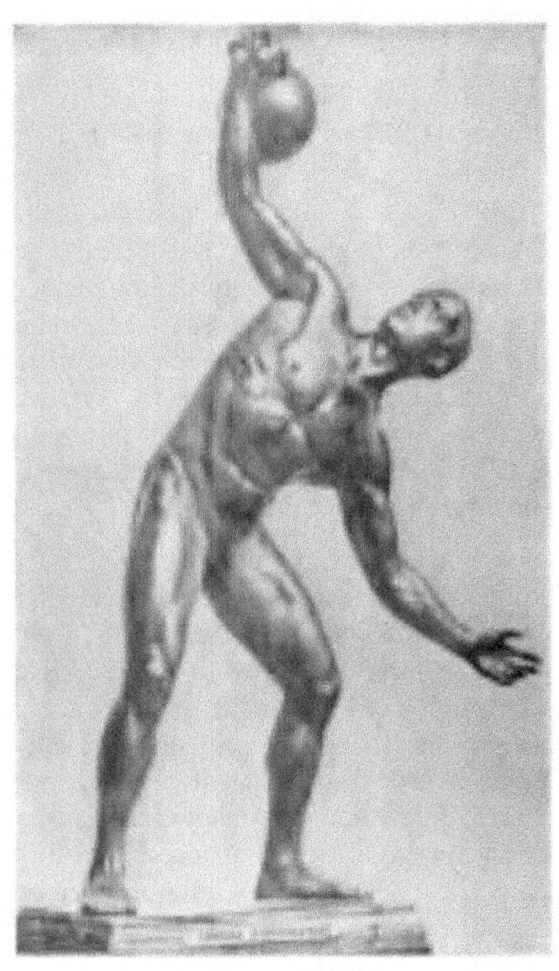

THE ATHLETE

A Statue in Bronze exhibited at the World's Fair in St. Louis

LIONEL STRONGFORT

A Brief Sketch

By LORD DOUGLAS, MARQUIS OF
QUEENSBERRY

TO those who contemplate taking a Course of Instruction to promote physical health and strength and to overcome, by natural methods, ailments and disorders, the chief consideration is always the selection of the most effective course to pursue. A good way and a very sane way to go about this would be to find out what qualifies the instructor who offers such a Course.

My connection with athletics and sports has led me to investigate many such methods of physical development. Of all the men I ever met, none impressed me so forcibly as Lionel Strongfort. His personality was forceful, sincerity was stamped in his words and action, and he showed the qualities that make a great teacher. I met him on many occasions, in America as well as in England, and came to appreciate the man more fully as I learned that back of all his efforts was not only a purpose to give to physical culture and all athletics the uplifting force of his own strong character, but to render also to the individual and to society a very real service.

From all I could learn, Strongfort was no different in youth from the ordinary boy, when his attention became fixed upon muscular development. From that period he began to seek out and reason why some men are stronger than others.

A Definite Aim In Life

THE more information he gathered the more his interest grew, until it resulted in a definite aim to develop strength in himself. Never, in his early years did he dream that he would eventually become known and recognized as the one human being nearest in approach to perfect symmetrical development.

His investigating; turn soon forced upon him the necessity of studying the human body and its organism. This opened to him the possibilities of overcoming defects in development, and he began to experiment just what movements strengthened the muscles and to seek a method by which every possible muscle in the human body could be gotten at in some way and strengthened and developed. It was not long before he found that Nature had laid down two rules that must be kept within in order to produce physical harmony, the first of these being diet and the second muscular activity.

THIS was the beginning of the theory that he afterward put in practice with so much success, for he realized that the perfectly strong man should not develop a few muscles at the expense of the others, but that physical perfection must mean strength in all parts of the body. Before long Lionel had outstripped youths of his age in feats of strength and this speedily extended to those older, larger and heavier than he was. Very naturally, he became known as being very strong and well developed and was much admired and commended by many because of his persistent application and the methodical way he pursued in proceeding to build up still greater strength and symmetry.

During this period Lionel did not neglect other duties, but, as he says, he found that he could apply himself more readily and absorb information more quickly the more he developed in health and strength.

When still in his teens Strongfort was induced to show his development and the ease with which he could handle heavy weights and bar-bells. He appeared before a private audience of many of the most prominent and distinguished people of New York City. His personal appearance and remarkable powers at once won for him the applause and friendship of many of those present and led to his making a professional engagement that took him first through all the principal theatres of this country and then across the water.

His Character Formed In Youth

It is a true indication of his character strength of purpose to note that in spite of becoming a world celebrity he has constantly continued with his teaching, just as at first he had made up his mind to do. From tile date of his first appearance before the general public, his time has been divided between personal instruction in physical and health culture, and public exhibition in the leading theatres of the world. This has brought him a world-wide reputation and a broad experience, which, coupled with his studies in Europe and America, has given him pre-eminence as an athlete and physical instructor.

At every performance he was accustomed to lifting, at arm's length above his head, with one hand, a bar-bell weighted to 312 pounds. This lift has never been equalled by any other athlete. In connection with this exhibition of strength there was a standing and widely advertised challenge to the world, together with an offer of a considerable sum of money, to the successful one who would duplicate the feat. Attempts were often made wherever Strongfort appeared, but no aspirant was ever successful.

An instance of the jealousy which actuates some of the athletic profession, is shown by an incident that happened during one of Strongfort's London engagements. Some provincial strong men who had made some notoriety in the small towns, thought out a clever trick to get a London engagement. The man and his confederate obtained access during the day to the stage of the theatre where Strongfort was performing. The shot used in the bar-bell to bring it to 312 lbs. weight was removed. When Strongfort, as was his nightly custom, invited anyone from the audience to lift the bar-bell, offering a prize therefore, this athlete from the provinces, stepped up and of course, could lift the much reduced bar-bell. It was a trying moment for Strongfort, who of course paid the reward. The trick was discovered, before the performance was closed, and the manager stepped forward and made an announcement to that effect. The strong man and his friend, however, had left the theatre.

An Unparalleled Test

PERHAPS one of his most remarkable performances is the automobile act. In this he supports upon his chest a bridge of 1,500 pounds in weight, over which is driven an automobile containing seven persons, the combined weight of bridge, automobile and passengers being approximately about 3/ tons. The suspension of this weight depends entirely upon the muscular strength of the performer. At the beginning of his experience several of his bones were broken, for the reason that he depended too much upon the strength of his bones. This, however, was entirely overcome when he learned to control and use his muscular development properly to fortify the bony frame to accomplish the feat.

This marvelous feat of Strength is done by Strongfort without the use of any blocks to support his back and knees, as is done by some inferior "strong man" who is faking some of the public which do not understand the difference.

He is the only man who has ever accomplished the tearing of five packs of playing cards at one time, a thickness of 260 cards. A part of his act was the lifting of a large basket bar-bell containing two men, each weighing upwards of 150 pounds; the turning of a back somersault with a 56-pound bell in each hand he accomplished with ease.

Strongfort is also an accomplished boxer, wrestler and bicycle racer and was engaged in almost every other variety of manly sport. His weight is about 180 pounds.

Louis Tuaillon, the noted Italian sculptor, was given a Governmental commission to model a statute in marble of Mr. Strongfort. This statue of heroic proportions is now in the National Art Gallery. Prof. Max Klinger, the European artist of marked ability and reputation, considered Strongfort the ideal of athletic symmetry and induced the athlete to pose for him. Several of this artist's pictures and statues, that arc considered masterpieces, are of the figure of Lionel Strongfort. The sculptor, Prof. Johannes Goetz, modeled a statue from Strongfort which work was com-pleted in bronze and exhibited at the St. Louis World's Fair.

I think I have met and come to know almost all the most famous athletes, and I have noted that Strongfort's remarkable strength and development has not been acquired at the expense of his health or vitality. He is in splendid condition, robust in health, full of endurance, stamina and energy. After more than five years had passed between two of our meetings, I found him, if anything, younger and more vigorous than ever in spite of a strenuous life of public exhibition and private teaching that only the exceptional man could endure. Undoubtedly, this is because he has always carefully and scientifically put into practice the results of his study covering physical training. He has developed a theory which he has rendered practical through personal practice and, as he puts it, those that follow his teachings have an example to guide them.

The Ideal Teacher

STRONGFORT expresses the ideal of the man who has achieved health and strength through endeavor. Not only can he duplicate his feats at any time, but exceed them. His vigor and vitality are pronounced, his robust healthfulness is refreshing to look upon. He is a deep thinker and student, given to research work. His knowledge of physiology, anatomy and hygiene is very broad and he is an advanced psychological scholar as well.

His extensive travels and living in close touch with all classes of people in almost every part of the civilized world enabled him to study their condition and requirements in their particular surroundings. Besides, his associations with the learned faculty of the many Universities and Colleges that he was called upon to visit, make him better fitted to teach the important subjects of Health and Strength Building, than anyone else 1 know of.

At the request of Dr. Dudley Sargent, of Harvard College, the demonstrations of Lionel Strongfort before the medical faculty were conducted to permit a practical study of the movements of all the visible muscles of the body, as well as to give a clearer insight into the results of development of internal muscular tissue upon the action of internal organs. The same series of demonstrations were also given at Brown University, Providence, R. I., and duplicated in the majority of the important seats of learning in Europe.

In commenting upon these demonstrations a scientist said:

"The rippling play of muscles under so perfect control not only portray the marvelous perfection to which the body can be developed, but forces upon us the realization of the wonderful structure given into our keeping and the folly of neglect and abuse of the same."

His Startling Discovery of Internal Muscular Development

It was only after some years of research, during which he made a close study of his pupils, in their physical change, that Strongfort made a startling announcement to the world. His patient work had led to the discovery that the maintenance of physical and mental health depended entirely upon the contractile power of the internal muscular structures. He found that weakness of the internal muscles invariably lead to displacement and functional disturbances. He proved, in his own person, that perfect health can be gained and maintained by the development of internal muscular strength and then he repeated this over and over again in the lives of his pupils. This is the principle upon which he founded the world-famous Strongfort methods. All of my medical friends were finally obliged to admit that Strongfort had found the Key to Normal Health. The efficient application of this fundamental principle has won for Strongfort a most unique position among the foremost benefactors of mankind.

His Unfailing Purpose

T'O his ambition, a most praiseworthy one in itself, he added a far higher purpose. He became conscious of a deeper purpose in nature—of the obligations he was under, and resolved to become a teacher and instructor of the method and system he perfected to gain his degree of health and strength. This resolution he has kept to the letter. There are more people scattered over the world to-day under his guidance and tuition than have ever been instructed by a single individual in the way of developing physical strength and health betterment.

In this little talk about Lionel Strongfort, I have not made any extravagant statements. Those who know him personally bear me out. In fact, I detest any ridiculous claims as arc made by press agents for some strong men, such as the biting of a chain, etc., which is absurd, and only calculated to hoodwink an unintelligent public. Any intelligent person knows that the material of the tooth is softer than iron and therefore cannot make an impression on iron. The evidence of the feats of strength of Lionel Strongfort is so well founded that there is not the slightest doubt attached to it, hence my endorsement. Also the evidence of his pupil graduates submitted to me prove his worthiness of their confidence and his ableness to guide and instruct rightly.

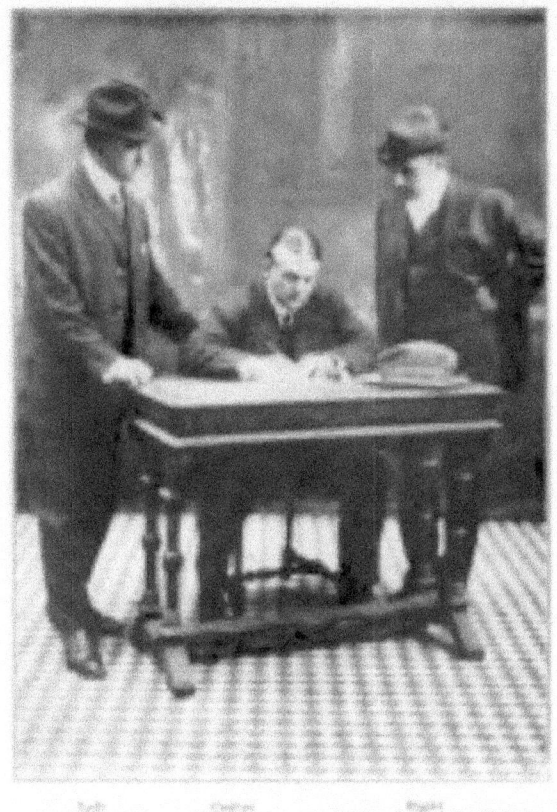

The Marquis of Queensberry

Signing His Endorsement of SPRINGFOOTISM

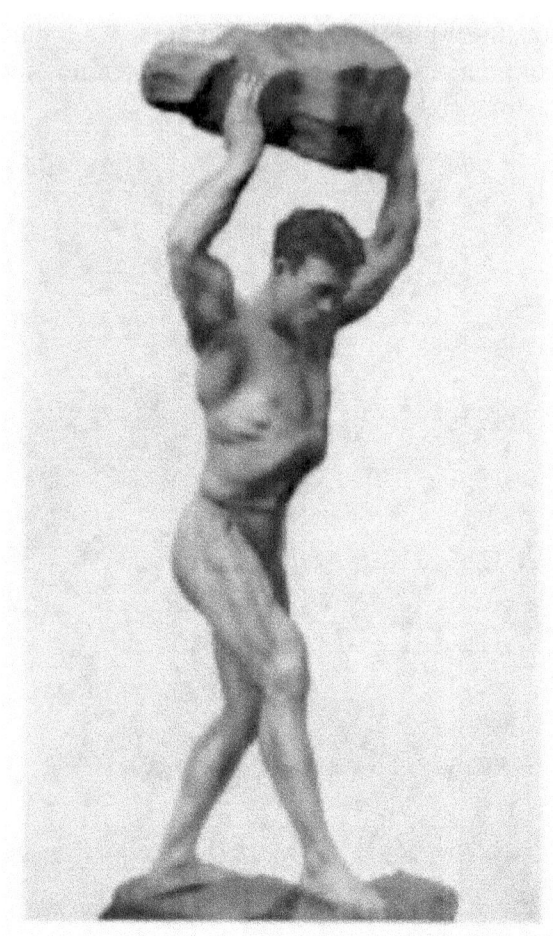

One of the many Sculptural poses of LIONEL STRONGFORT

Physical Vigor and Success

T'HIS is an age in which intelligence is at a premium. Brain is often said to be more important than brawn. But in looking at the importance of brain ttto closely, one loses the perspective and is likely to overlook the fact that both brain and brawn are necessary for all purposes.

Men of brains these days make a careful study of the problems of success in life and its requirements. And. the really intelligent man soon comes to see that achievement depends as much upon physical vigor and robust health as upon unusual qualities of mind. Most of our great men have been men of unusual physical energy, possessing the most hardy and powerful constitutions. They have developed such strength of body and of nerve in youth that they retain their vigor almost for a lifetime. The great importance of Physical Fitness is recognized by men of highest authority the world over.

There are thousands of men of exceptional ability who might be successful, but who fail because of the lack of constitutional strength. Real health does not mean the ability to sit up and walk around a bit, and to cat breakfast with the aid of a drug store. Real health means unlimited vitality. It means the capacity for endless work, without feeling tired. It means exuberant spirits. It means a pleasing, forceful and magnetic personality. It means a clear head and an active mind. It means that one realizes all his possibilities.

To understand this so as to apply it to the perfect control of the body—this is the Science of Strongfortism, which I have popularized and brought within the understanding of all, so that it could be applied by the individual with perfect success, whatever the physical ailment may be.

Mental Power vs. Mind and Will

YOUR natural capacities are what you make them. No matter what abilities or talents you possess, your mental powers will be greatly multiplied by increased physical vigor. If you are a common-place and uninteresting individual because of your lack of health, you may become a distinct, magnetic personality by developing your latent powers. It can be done. Some of my pupils have made amazing progress in business after the awakening that follows an intimate, personal Course of Instruction under my guidance. The physical life is fundamental, and your mental and moral qualities, together with your strength of will, or lack of will power, will depend upon your physical stances.

Life is a struggle for achievement, or it is a vegetable existence. If you are not a success, then it is time for you to think hard. Have you strong nerves, poise and the ability to master any emergency, or do you get shaky in time of excitement? Have you the initiative to go ahead and act, or only do what you are told? Are you on top, or are you the under dog? In the battle of life, are you struggling in self-defence, in unconscious acknowledgement of your weakness, or are you fighting on the offensive with a strong, confident and courageous hand.

Double Your Chance of Success

TO double your strength and energy means more than doubling your chance of success. It means multiplying your chances of success a hundred or a thousand times. Just as in a race, even if you are losing first, to double your speed would not merely double your chances, but would multiply them a thousand times, and make it absolutely certain that you would win.

In life, to be a success or a failure, to accomplish something or to accomplish anything, is to BE something or to BE nothing. Which do you choose? It is up to you. You can choose either way. If you choose to be something and to do something, then begin at the bottom and build the foundation upon which everything else depends. It is not a question of being born right; it is a question of making the most of yourself with the facilities that have been given you. Every man has the capacity for success in some direction if he will make the most of himself. It is for you to choose whether you will be a man of power or a weakling.

What You Owe to Others

IT is your duty to your parents to make the most of yourself. It is your duty to your wife and children, if you have or ever will have a wife and little ones. It is your duty to the world, to humanity in general. And most of all, it is your duty to yourself. Make up your mind to be the greatest success that is possible with your faculties at their best. Determine that you will have that constitutional strength, that vitality, that untiring nervous energy, and the clear, active brain, without which success is impossible.

"No man can win in the battle of life who has not COURAGE and PERSISTENCY. And as neither of these are found where ENERGY is lacking, it must follow that ENERGY is THE indispensable quality of GREAT SUCCESS."

Delusion of Health Without Strength

STRENGTH is an absolute essential in securing and maintaining any normal degree of health. There are those who, themselves lacking in muscular vigor, are prone to speak contemptuously of the same, declaring that what they desire is not great "ugly" muscles, but just health! It occasionally happens also that some weakling will declare that he is in perfect health, inasmuch as he is out of bed and able to walk around.

But, as a matter of fact, no one can enjoy a high degree of health unless he represents a high standard of physical vigor. He should be a good specimen of animal life. And th:s means that he must be at least normally strong. What would we think of the health of a horse or dog that was not thoroughly alive with active energetic muscles?

Normally, muscle makes up nearly one-half of the bulk of the human body, or almost three times as much as any other tissue or part. The greater part of our food is required to maintain the muscles and repair the cell life that is constantly being used up; and two-thirds of our vital heat is produced by muscular activity.

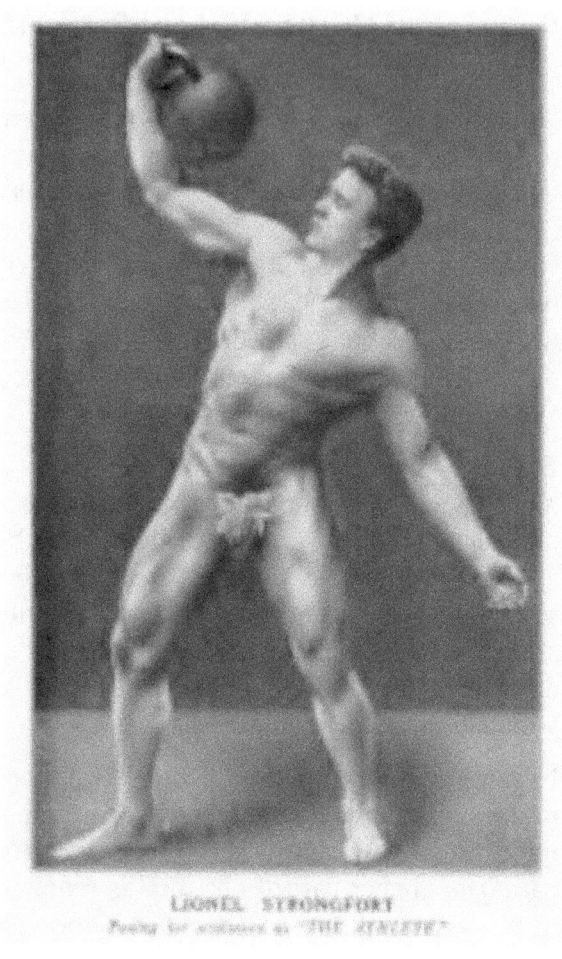

LIONEL STRONGFORT
Posing for sculptors as "THE ATHLETE"

For good health, therefore, it is important that muscle should constitute at least forty-three per cent, of the entire body, and that this tissue should be in the very best condition. A good circulation depends absolutely upon sufficient active exercise for these muscles, as does also the proper action of all the vital and functional organs, which readily lose vigor without the tonic effect of such exercise. In the human body, as throughout all Nature, activity is the law of life, whereas stagnation means decay and ultimate death. How absurd, therefore, the notion that physical frailty may be consistent with good health. It is not sufficient that one should eat carefully, enjoy pure air or even breathe deeply. One must be STRONG, with the stamina and strength of manhood, or with the vigor of robust womanhood.

Drugs and Dopes Are Dangerous

YOU cannot obtain health and strength by the use of tonics, stimulants, drugs, laxatives or purgatives—in liquid, tablet, pill or any other form. The physician of experience and knowledge will tell you how impotent such means are toward effecting a permanent cure. Medicines may relieve a situation by stimulating organic functions, but such stimulus coming from unnatural causes, may do more harm than good. Nature is the real restorer, the real creator, the real healer, the real cure. If a condition of constipation exists, the administration of a cathartic or some such physic may remove the obstruction in the bowels, but it does not cure the constipated habit.

There is no greater menace to the physical condition than to be constantly taking pills or tablets, either to relieve pain or to prevent constipation. It is dangerous to be under the influence of the various patent "remedies" with which the market is unfortunately flooded. You must adopt Nature's method. If you have violated Nature's laws it is to Nature you must apply for pardon. And Nature casts a decided frown on all such methods of filling your stomach with chemical concoctions, sometimes of doubtful combinations. There never yet was a man who regained health and strength and vitality by pampering his stomach, and there never will be, either. Common, ordinary intelligence, will tell you that pills, potions and other similar piffle are in most cases inventions of quacks to separate the honest searcher for health from his hard-earned money, and to keep up the delusion that the only way to attain health is by consuming enough of it. Artificial methods never have produced, and never will produce any lasting results, and to attempt to attain them by any such means is a dangerous and usually disastrous risk that no one can afford to run. STRONGFORTISM is based on NATURAL laws and STRONGFORTISM has never known a failure.

You Are Not Too Old

IF you are one of those who think they are too old, think it no longer. Physical activity should be continued to the very end. When one reaches the point at which such activity is utterly impossible, then, truly, he is only a step from the end.

It is commonly supposed that weakening and stiffening of the body is the result of age, but it would be nearer the truth to say that age is the result of a weakening and stiffening of the muscles. Youth is a period of activity, and one can retain youth only by continuing such activity. Some of the most remarkable athletic feats of endurance have been accomplished by so-called old men—old in years, but young in condition.

Scientific exercise is even more important for men and women past 40 or 50 years of age than for their sons and daughters. The considerations previously mentioned upon the subject of complete versus incomplete movements apply with particular force to those who have passed the elastic years of youth. The many years of incomplete movements in the daily affairs of life have gradually limited the action possibilities of their muscles and stiffened them as well, and in order to retain health and youth up to their declining days it is especially necessary that they should take regular exercise of a kind to preserve elasticity as well as the strength of their muscles.

What You Owe To Yourself

TO develop and maintain the highest degree of physical perfection that is possible is your duty. We hear a good deal about the necessity for thrift, for saving money, but we hear so little about the necessity of thrift in health, of saving and building up a reserve force of energy. A moment's thought will convince you which is the better. When I travel about and study the people whom I meet, I am amazed at the utter disregard of personal physical appearance which is so common everywhere.

How much different the whole world might be if each man and woman had the desire to bring about as great a physical perfection as possible! When next you sec a well developed, healthy man or woman, try to think what a different place this might be if there were more people of that standard.

Physical Fitness—The Greatest Asset

PERSONAL appearance is more than fifty per cent, of a man's assets. If he applies for a position, and nine hundred and ninety-nine in the thousand are doing this all the time, his physical makeup is either for or against him at the first glance.

An employer can investigate a man's business record, but he can't investigate his physical condition. A man must carry this with him always as prima facie evidence of his soundness and right living. With such assets to begin with, a business man is justified in going further, but without it, nine times in ten he is satisfied that the applicant cannot fill the position because of his physical appearance.

That the majority of people are not better physically than they are is due more to the individual than to outward causes. It is true with many there have been extenuating circumstances, but can you honestly say that such is your case? Ask yourself honestly, if your present position is not due more to your own neglect than to anything else.

You know that it is not what you eat so much as how; it- is not so much what you do, what activity or exercise you follow; but how. Your functional activity depends upon your physical activity. When these two are in harmony, when you are eating, sleeping and bathing rightly, and then bringing about a perfect organic functioning of your whole body, your physical and mental powers will be brought up to their highest efficiency.

Many persons recognize their deficiencies and yet never give time nor thought to correcting them. Or, they promise themselves they will do something—tomorrow— unmindful of the fact that the crack thief of Time, Mr. Procrastinator, will steal to the last minute of existence, and leave the victim, the putter-off, a doddering, decrepit failure, dependent on others, haunted by the memories of countless "meant-to-do" promises. If one knows there is a way to such correction and does not take advantage of that way, it is a still worse condemnation of self-neglect, for if people do not know, they are not so much to be blamed. That is why I am so persistently trying to make known the light, the truth, to those who still do not know. The provoking, the unreasonable part of it all is with those who do realize their own physical deficiencies and their mental poverty, and yet will not lift a hand to lift themselves out of the rut.

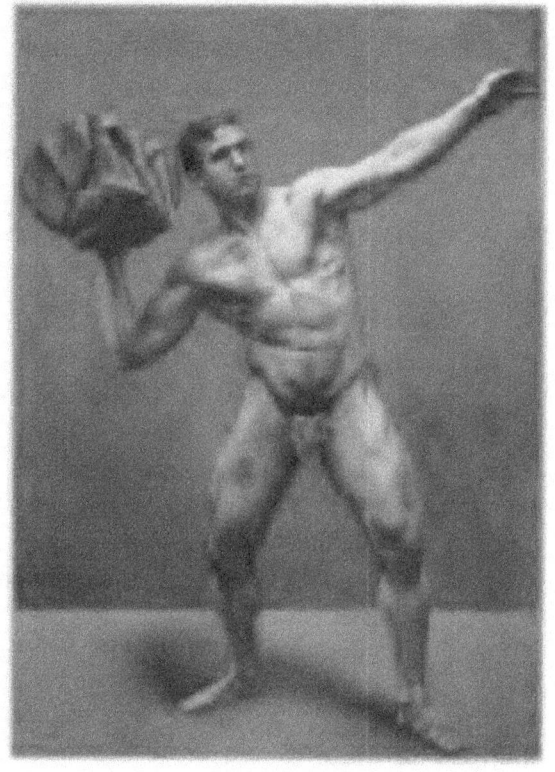

Another Sculptor Study of LIONEL STRONGFORT

Are You Worth Saving?

TO be thin, run-down, stoop-shouldered, flat-chested and emaciated is a direct reflection upon the character in many ways. It may mean not sufficient intelligence to know anything about the care of the body. This is something that it should not be possible to say of any man or woman, and this is another reason why I am working so hard to spread intelligence in regard to physical and health development.

If such is not the case, it may then reflect that there is a willful neglect of the health and the body. There is a still more serious matter, for, even though you do not consider yourself of sufficient value to be worth building up so that you can get the fullest earning power of your natural capacity, yet from the point of view of merely saving yourself bodily suffering and mental anguish, and the chance of making yourself a burden upon others, you should at least make an effort to secure such safety.

Self-neglect not only means danger to you, but it means that you become a menace to others. The welfare of the whole of society says this must not be so, and constantly laws are being enacted to compel men and women to live and act rightly.

Do not let it be said of you that your appearance shows either ignorance of the proper care of your body or carelessness and neglect of what should be your most precious possession in this life—your body—since it is the basis of all your happiness and success.

The world will take you at your own estimate of yourself, remember. It is self-evident that men who consider their bodies of little value will be on just such a corresponding plane in the estimation of others, as it is only fair to suppose that negligence of the body means negligence in all else.

Intelligence in Physical and Health Promotion

The Necessity For Care In Training

ATTEMPTED physical and health promotion without intelligent direction and a thorough knowledge of the body and its needs may be physical destruction rather than any true development. There are many who fancy that they need no special knowledge in order to become strong and vigorous, but that if they merely exercise in some way or another the results will come. It is true that such methods arc sometimes of benefit, but on the other hand also it is often detrimental.

This fact accounts for the superiority of Strongfortism in giving results. A pupil is always under my personal care and it is this intelligent direction of all his efforts which adds both interest during such instruction and ultimate success.

The novice, struggling blindly to get strong, is apt to make all manner of mistakes in his ignorance. When dealing with vitality no one can afford to experiment. The fact that there are thousands who have attempted some form of physical improvement without proper guidance, and who have signally failed to accomplish such improvement, is evidence of just as great a need for definite knowledge and a competent teacher in connection with physical education as in connection with the development of the mind.

The Dangers of Over-Training

ONE of the most serious evils associated with unintelligent effort is the danger of over-training. Exercise should never be too violent or too prolonged. When such exercise is carried out excessively or in any way indulged to an extreme degree it produces an undue excitability of the heart and sometimes causes it to become enlarged. There is a form of heart trouble induced by this over-exertion which sets up a degenerating influence upon that organ, causing it to lose its vigor and muscular power.

The heart, being an involuntary muscle, responds to its service regardless of the volition of the person, and an increase of work put upon it by this excess of exercise results in this disorder. It is a very common trouble, even in persons whose occupations are very laborious and to which they are exposed for too long a period. At no stage, whatever the age, is it wise to endeavor to promote health and strength by unwisely undertaking too much exercise or training.

I cannot emphasize too strongly the great advantages, both in safety and accomplishments of having always a Teacher of the highest experience, in whom you can place implicit confidence.

Faith, you know, moves mountains. I would have you acquire the faith of Hajnos, the famous Hercules of the U. S. Navy. When he first wrote to me he was a weakling, with all the frailties of a Gob (he said so frankly when he enrolled) he said:

"I place my faith wholly in you, my teacher, to bring me back to health and physical vigor, and I will live up to your teachings faithfully."

If you will give me that kind of faith, I can promise you big things, too, in achievement. Over-training undermines the health just as any other form of overwork. It is more destructive because of the rapid consumption of vitality if one trains beyond a certain point. It is important, therefore, to know how much to exercise as to know how it should be done and when the proper amount is taken that is necessary to bring about increased development and maintain perfect health.

Misconceptions About Bodily Activity

IT is important that some very wrong impressions held by people should be corrected. There is a certain class who like to try and show what they think is a superior knowledge, by laughing at physical culturists. In this, however, he who laughs last laughs best.

This kind of person believes that because lie has two legs, and can move about, eat his meals regularly and hold down some kind of a job, there is nothing the matter with him. He very glibly recommends good, honest work as a sufficient means of building muscular tissue and promoting bodily vigor. The folly of this, however, is obvious, even to those who have never given the subject any special study, for among the millions of workers of the world there are very few who can claim anything like a symmetrical or athletic development.

Nearly all forms of labor are such as to overwork certain parts of the body while neglecting the muscles of other parts. But, in addition to the one-sided development thus brought about, most forms of manual work arc of an exhausting character; they consume, but do not build strength; they drain one's vitality, stiffen his joints and make him angular and slow.

Why did you go to school? To train and develop your mind. Why not train and develop your body? Because one learned to read enough to follow the comic pages, it does not follow by any means that such was the limit of capacity to learn. Many things may have stood between a youth in grammar school, and a college education or a career of fame. Not the least of these may have been the failure to train the body at the same time, and in the same degree as the mind.

First Of All Be Square With Yourself

NOTHING but your own sinful weakness of body and your lack of the initial strength to make the first step toward your physical education, can be blamed. This is a free country. No one can make you do something against your will. If you cannot be square enough, honest enough with yourself to bring out the best that is in you, then you must stay where you arc.

It is true that there are a few varieties of "honest toil" which might be physically beneficial to any one, but the prevailing long hours for work more than offset the good results that might accrue in such cases, and the fact remains that most laborers are sadly lacking in any true bodily culture. Even to the working man, scientific physical training is as much a necessity as to anyone else.

It is a remarkable fact that I have a very large enrollment of pupils who are farmers. They write me from all parts of the world. Now, here is a class of workers, living almost wholly an outdoor life, and from daylight to dark engaged strenuously in often very laborious work. Their need of a balancing activity is evident from the fact that so many of the more intelligent farmers seek my help and learn the way to right living and a fuller, happier life than they ever knew before.

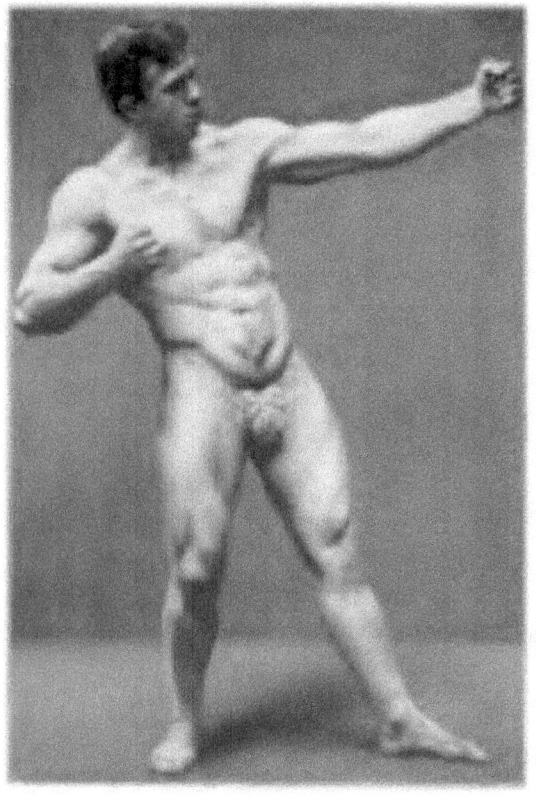

Another Sculptural Study of LIONEL STRONGFORT.
"THE DISCUS"

The face and torso are modeled for the title in a clear instant of the body.

Women and Housework

IN the case of women, especially, these remarks apply with great force, in spite of the fact that general housework has been repeatedly, though mistakenly, recommended as a form of beneficial exercise. If only a limited amount of it is done, and that energetically, there may be some physical benefits, but the wrecked and shapeless figures of millions of housewives throughout the entire civilized world, after a number of years of domestic work, stand out as incontestable evidence that housework cannot take the place of systematic exercise.

Athletic Games Insufficient

AGAIN, there are those who fancy that games and athletic sports will take the place of rational, systematic training. The writer certainly should be the last to object to games and, athletic sports of any kind; indeed, he practices and advocates them warmly. But in the majority of cases they are far from sufficient to answer all requirements in the way of uniform and symmetrical development, or even of that strength and vigor which are necessary in the games themselves. An athletic pastime, like some special form of work, usually involves the use of certain muscles or sets of muscles at the expense of others, and the result is an uneven development. Whoever is familiar with athletes is also familiar with the fact that a large majority of them are far from symmetrical or well built. They are round-shouldered more often than otherwise. As a usual thing, the athlete who specializes in some particular branch of sport is to blame for his one-sided build. Strictly speaking, such a man is not truly an athlete, for he is incapable of anything but his specialty.

What Makes The Real Athlete?

THE true athlete, first of all, should be perfectly built in every part, and therefore should be capable of creditable participation in any and all branches of athletics, including feats of actual strength, wrestling, boxing, running, jumping, weight throwing and all other popular pastimes. Special systematic exercises for all parts of the body are necessary to perfect the athlete, even for his best success in athletics, and it is a fact that the wisest and the most successful athletes, when in training, depend largely upon the use of special movements for each individual part of the body, in addition to the practice of their athletic specialty. No one should attempt any strenuous athletic effort until he has made himself fit by special training of the entire body.

Symmetrical Development

BUT if mere games are not sufficient for full and complete development, the same must be said of many forms of physical training actually designed for all-round development. Thousands may be found who have depended, not upon athletics, but upon regular exercise, who are yet far from symmetrical. Some of the most round-shouldered young men that I have ever seen have been among those trained for some years on the usual gymnasium apparatus, including horizontal and parallel bars, flying rings, ladders, vaulting horses, rubber strand apparatus, and the rest.

It is true that such apparatus offers one advantage, that of stimulating interest in the work, but this frequently carries with it the disadvantage of developing some parts of the body at the expense of another. The "gym" enthusiast sometimes develops a splendid set of arms and shoulders, to the neglect of his legs and the lower part of the torso. And outside of the gymnasium there are many other examples of unequal proportion in physique, ranging from the track athlete, who is all legs, to the wrestler, who is all neck and arms, or the fellow who demonstrates the use of the new fangled exercises made of rubber strands. These are often to be seen in store windows, where the demonstration is made to try and sell the apparatus. The man using them of course shows a big arm and chest development, and the unthinking observer might be impressed with the great show of muscle, forgetting the fact that even a boot-black gets much the same arm and chest muscles by reason of moving the arms back and forth.

Experiments Are Costly

THE teaching of physical fitness is still in a more or less experimental stage, which accounts for the frequency with which those seeking health and strength by instruction from physical culture teachers are so often disappointed, for the reason that these instructors or teachers are not themselves qualified in the science of health and body building.

It is true, they have a smattering of this knowledge and possibly are honest in their opinion that they have commendable systems, but their systems are not sufficiently thorough, nor do they begin at the proper point and systematically and methodically build upward, as ought to be done. In other words, the majority of these teachers do not comprehend the requirements of the body, and therefore cannot take into consideration the many factors that are essential in the ideal plan of physical betterment and health promotion.

Such teachers aim to get attention by their bombastic advertising methods, hoping to create a big impression by their claims, and so hoodwink the public.

"Unnatural" Systems of Training

ONE of the first requirements of any rational method of training is that it should be thoroughly natural, or, in other words, in harmony with the structure and normal usage of the different parts of the body. But in many cases the most unnatural measures and devices are used for bringing about results. In some instances, also, the development is "forced" along by measures which are ever and ever a little beyond the powers of the body to respond to readily.

Such forcing methods are unnatural. It would be far more to the pupil's advantage and welfare if he were allowed to progress more slowly, but in a more natural way. Indeed, the ultimate result would be a greater degree of strength as a result of the more moderate and more natural development. Nature must be considered in these as in other matters, for no man can disregard or violate her laws without paying the penalty.

Complete versus Incomplete Movements

A serious fault with some devices and forms of exercise is that they do not afford "complete" movements, or, in other words, movements which bring a muscle into play throughout the full reach in which it is capable of acting. This is particularly true where rubber strands or steel springs are used. The same objection applies to many games, which, despite their undoubted value, are not ample for all of the physiological requirements of exercise. Only by "complete" movements can the muscles be kept pliable and elastic, or even as uniformly strong as they should be.

It may be interesting to note that the chief necessity for special forms of exercise is due to the fact that in the daily affairs and activities of life the most of our movements are of the "incomplete" character; even such muscles as are called into action from time to time, being employed in short, jerky, limited movements, involving only a short segment of the arc through which the affected member may be carried in a complete movement. When one's exercise, like the ordinary affairs of life, has to do only with movements of this character, a more or less muscle-bound condition is usually the result. It is essential, therefore, that exercise should afford not only plenty of action, but the maximum of action for each and every part.

For this reason, among others, various lifting and stretching machines are very, very far from being adapted for general use.

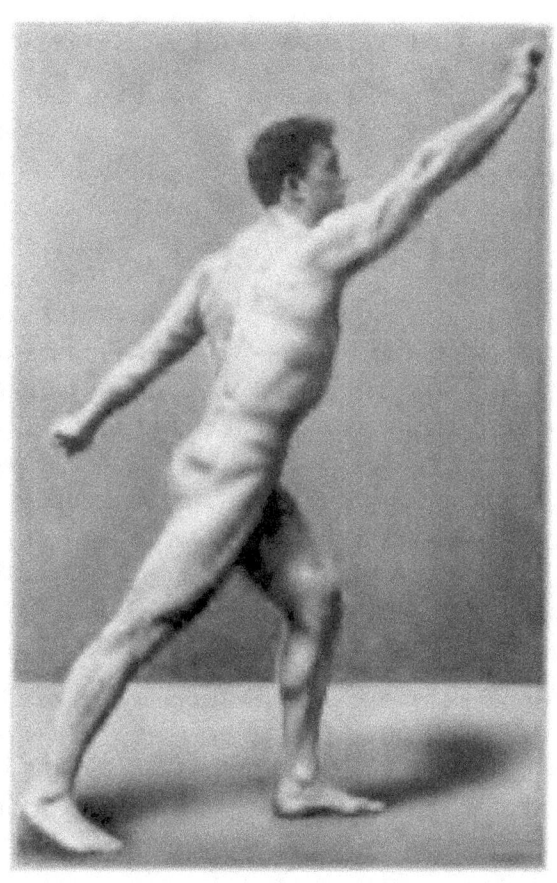

A Profile Pose

Showing the Remarkable Symmetry of STRONGFORT'S Figure

Muscle Contraction Systems

VERY similar objections apply to a number of systems of so-called exercise without apparatus, classified generally under the heads of tensing and vibratory exercises. Some of the vendors of these exercise lessons, sometimes called evolutions, make extravagant claims for their system upon alleged psychological grounds, claiming to have discovered some weird and mysterious connection between mind and muscle which had never been understood before and which will enable one to gain far greater strength — just as if will power or mental determination may not be brought into play to an equal or greater extent by any other.

The above objections to incomplete movements apply with special force to the vibratory exercises and the tensing movements. They also have the muscle-binding and stiffening tendencies. It is doubtful if any muscular strength can be acquired in this way. The muscles are not developed naturally, only exercised. The essence of such exercise is the resistance of one muscle or set of muscles against another, the entire limb or other member thus being made tense and rigid. So that instead of the various muscles of the body being brought individually under control, and trained to act harmoniously with each other, they are simply trained to antagonize each other.

Danger of Heart Strain

THE possibilities for mental concentration, furthermore, when desirable, are all in favor of other more natural systems of exercise. For the boasted use of "will-power" in connection with the tensing movements can avail nothing, because in the very nature of the exercise the effort (or mental effort, if you prefer) can never be concentrated upon one single muscle, but must be divided between that muscle and the other muscle which is required

The claim frequently made in connection with these tensing or "antagonistic" exercises, to the effect that while they offer as much resistance as the use of heavy weights, yet they do not strain the heart in the same way, is sheer nonsense on the face of it. To secure the same resistance with the antagonistic exercices, the strain upon the heart is just twice as great, for there is double the effort and twice as many muscles are used in the same exercise. Of the two methods, the actual use of heavy weights is the more natural, the more effective and safer.

Heavy Weightlifting

THE practice of heavy weight-lifting, however, is not to be recommended for the average man in search of health and strength. Before he begins such practice he must be prepared through a preliminary course of light resistant weight-, so that his muscular system is well fortified for the heavier task about to be imposed upon it. If you arc interested in heavy weight-lifting feats of strength and superior development, you should read my book, "The Strength of a Hercules." I will send it on request.

Spinal Adjustments

MECHANICAL adjustments of the vertebrae of the spine by manual pressure, cannot be of permanent benefit unless proper steps are taken to symmetrically develop the adjacent muscular structures upon which the normal position of the spine is dependent. Thus it becomes necessary to have one or more adjustments made each week because, while it is possible to force displaced or "slipped" vertebrae back into normal position, the deficiency of the attending muscles will cause another "slip," and then another adjustment is required.

All of this expensive procedure will be unnecessary for those who adopt a Course of Strongfortism, for it is always my purpose to include with every Course sufficient instruction for the symmetrical development and strengthening of the muscular structures associated with the spine. When this natural condition has been restored, harmonious action of these muscles will retain the vertebrae in normal position.

The principles of Strongfortism embody all that is logical and re ultful in the building of Health, Strength and Sexual Vigor and the correction of anatomical defects. All of this priceless knowledge, once obtained places your health, happiness, all your future business success within your own

Danger of Rubber Strands

THERE have been many kinds of physical culture apparatus put on the market. Few, if any, have any merits that recommend them above well proved gymnasium equipment. The present use by tome of the so- called physical culture instructors of the old-fashioned rubber strand exerciser shows how slow some of them are to make progress. I can remember many years ago seeing in the old dime museum on 14th Street, a little, but unsymmetrical foreign, freak Strongman, practicing with such rubber strand apparatus attached to a board on which he stood. This man was interested in selling the apparatus which he offered with a little booklet for about a dollar. It is sad to reflect in our day, that some self-styled physical culture instructors arc not only still using that antiquated and inefficient apparatus, but claiming it as their invention. The same holds good in regard to the rubber strand exerciser now offered, attached to handles, and which were known many years ago as chest expanders and could be bought in any sporting goods store for a dollar or so.

It is wrong to use such rubber strand apparatus for many reasons. They are dangerous. The handles may slip from the fingers. The strands may snap and injure, in so doing, the face or eyesight. But the most important objection is that the muscular action is limited only to the extent of the stretching of the rubber which also can be done only in one direction. Thus only a few muscles can be exercised which are over-developed at the expense of others

Another objection is that the pull of the muscles is not uniform, the resistance of the rubber increasing as stretched, whereas the resistance should be uniform throughout the complete muscular movement.

After all is said, it remains that a scientific dumb-bell such as the Strongfort Resistance-Increasing, remains the one perfect and ideal exercise apparatus because of the principle of graduated increase of resistance which it affords and this resistance remaining the same through each muscular movement, and every muscle of the body can be uniformly exercised.

The Yeast Fad

I feel that I should devote a few words to the yeast fad, which manufacturers are trying to promote the consumption of, by making extravagant claims for its use as a bowel corrective. This simply places it in the same category as drugs

Now in order to justify their claim for yeast, they advocate in their literature that primarily diet and exercise are fundamental principles in promoting health and regulating bowel action. Then, why bother with yeast, when diet and exercise are the first essential, and they secure the ends in themselves?

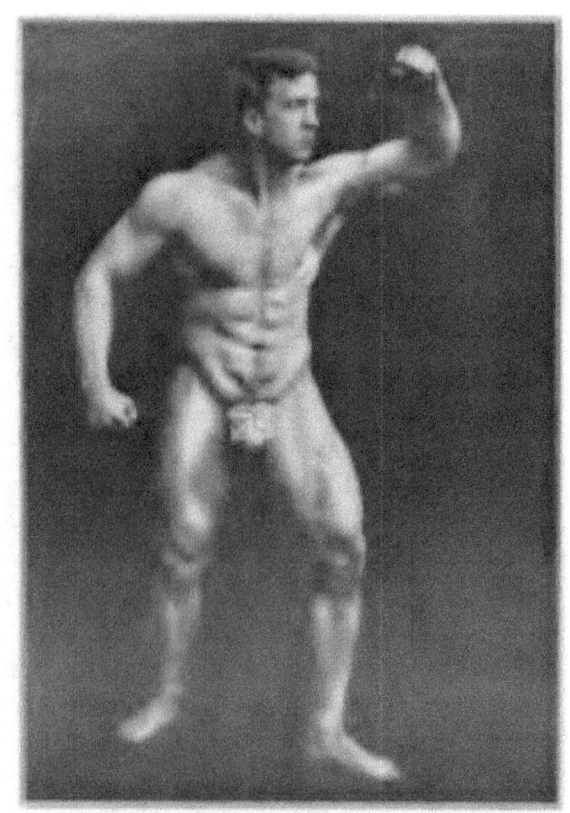

STRONGFORT'S Famous Gladiator Pose

Should and Jujitsu are omitted to avoid hiding the muscular outline.

Strongfortism

The Science of Promoting Physical Fitness through
Internal and External Muscular Harmony.

STRONGFORTISM expresses the essence
and guiding principle of what it teaches—
fundamental health and strength. There is no
vagueness and mystery here. Nothing which
is beyond and above the understanding of
every day common reasoning—Uniform
strength embodies health —there can be no
such strength without health. Wherever there
is internal as well as external strength, there
must be health. Whenever organic strength is
impaired the health is also. We can reverse
this and say, whenever health is impaired,
strength decreases. Health and strength arc
inseparable. The balance between them is
maintained by muscular activity. Whenever
some transgression of Nature's laws affect
them, we must turn to Nature for restoration.

Nature is never at rest. She is constant in her
endeavor —creating, building, destroying in
her process of evolution. Nature is active, and
activity is life. Rest, complete rest, is
impossible. If there is not growth, then there
must be decay. Movement there must be,
forward to greater perfection, to higher
purposes and usefulness, or backward, to

dissolution. In our tranquil repose or sleep, Nature is ever rebuilding, restoring—extend this period beyond the time required by Nature and she will stop in her work of restoration and allow degenerating influences to begin their sway toward decrease and decay.

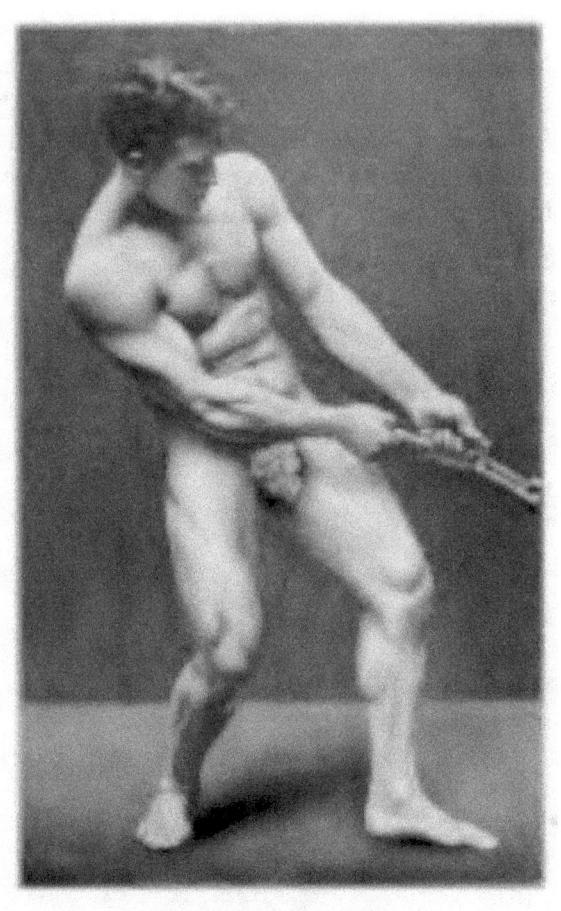

LIONEL STRONGFORT

From the Amazing Strength and Herculid Power in this Pose

Every Ailment Is Overcome

STRONGFORTISM in its practice covers the requirements of every person—man or woman, young or old, sick or well. It teaches the care of the body necessary to overcome disorder and ailment and to promote health.

Whatever the physical ailment may be, there will be found in the instruction planned to fit that case, precise, and particular information that applies specifically to such trouble. It will be so clear and easily understood and put into practice by the pupil that almost immediate results are noticeable.

So true are the principles to Nature's requirements and yet so easily applied, that even with the first lesson very marked benefits are noticeable.

It teaches how to develop health and to recover health, and with health an increase of strength. It practically and thoroughly instills scientific activity of the muscular system; it promotes the co-ordination of activity throughout the body—the muscular tissue is rendered flexible, resilient, firm in texture, strong in fibre, the nervous system energized, the mental faculties stimulated.

Why Results Are Obtained

THE first step toward this end is bringing into play every muscle of the body, external and internal, for these reasons:

First: Because scientific activity as taught by Strong- fortism exerts a more consistent and powerful influence upon health and life than any medicinal agent known to science. The very first improvement is noticeable by the better functional performance of the organs of the body, whose duty it is to throw off the poisonous waste material which has accumulated and clogged the system and given rise to ailment, disorder and disease.

Second: Because methodical scientific activity brings into play the muscles that bear upon the action of the internal organs upon which depend the digestive processes. The food is assimilated better and more nutrition obtained to rebuild the wasted tissue in muscle and organ.

Third: Because scientific activity, practically applied, produces a better circulation of the blood, which deposits the nutriment with which it is enriched, in every portion of the body, muscular tissue, nerve cells and brain substance.

Fourth: Because scientific activity increases the capacity of the lungs to purify the blood and make it more capable of sustaining life and nourishing the tissues. Remember that every organ of the body is subservient to the others, yet each has its own office to perform. Scientific activity means functional activity in every organ. It develops the strength and power in the entire system to resist and to overcome disease.

With the scientific methods as employed in Strongfortism, an active combat against the disease in evidence takes place at once, and the system is so invigorated that it eradicates all danger of any other disease that may be lurking in the human body. Strongfortism fortifies against all ills, present and future, by transforming the body into such a healthy, natural, normal condition that disease cannot live in it. The means employed are natural, the benefits received are natural, and for this reason Strongfortism is an abiding and complete success.

The Source of Mental Power

STRONGFORTISM in its scientific activity increases the mental power, develops the mind and strengthens the will. Not only is mental activity dependent upon vital activity in the brain, but development of the brain is dependent upon the supply of blood. The growth of the intellect requires the same process as the building of muscular tissue; activity to destroy the worn cells, and nutriment to supply with living, vital material. The mind is the product of the brain. There can be no strength of mind; there can be no will; no intelligence, even, without brain substance.

The mind gives us the ability to perceive sensations, to be conscious, to exercise reason and judgment, and to will, in accordance to what our reason and judgment dictates. Physical exercise is a demand that Nature makes upon us in order to promote and maintain health. The exercise of the mind in an unhealthy body further weakens and debilitates that body, because it exhausts the vitality by drawing upon the nutrition to supply the material to build up the waste brain substance, brought about by mental activity.

Bodily derangement produces mental derangement, brain fag, mental fatigue, lack of concentration, inability to produce.

Mental inefficiency is not wholly the result of mental application, but more often the result of insufficient bodily health. A proportional physical development will produce mental development for the reason that the body, having all the organs functioning properly, can supply the nutriment for the muscular tissues and supply, at the same time, the nutrition demanded by the brain that is developing in its sphere of activity.

A good memory is the insignia of a healthy brain and body. When the memory begins to fail it is an indication of failing physical powers. Increased physical power invigorates the brain and strengthens the memory, just as it increases the capacity of the mind and produces a moral courage that makes itself known by exertion of the will in overcoming and resisting influences that degrade.

Promotes Business Success

PHYSICAL poise is then the outgrowth of health and strength. Mental poise is the reflection of a healthy brain produced by a healthy body. Both are acquired through the attainment of health and strength. Strongfortism promotes health and strength in the highest

The brain, like the body, requires periods of relaxation. Continuous activity acts upon the brain as it does upon the muscular system, causing too great depletion of the cells. When exercised scientifically and in moderation, the physical system rebounds, acquiring more strength and vigor and vitality and accelerated activity; so does the brain.

When the brain becomes fatigued, therefore, it requires relaxation and recreation. This is well afforded by exercises of a physical character. Aside from being refreshed and repaired by the usual night's repose that comes to the brain and body, physical and mental recuperation are strongly promoted by suitable exercise. Remember, mental endeavor, mental force, mental energy, can best be cultivated and sustained when the physical side is also cultivated and promoted in health and strength; and it is injurious to attempt to cultivate the brain and mind at the expense of the body. First and foremost, to attain mental efficiency, physical health and strength must be obtained through scientific activity.

The most pronounced benefits are obtained through the practice of Strongfortism in promoting greater mental efficiency. This is confirmed repeatedly by the greater business success and increased earning power acquired by so many Strongfort Pupils.

The Importance of Diet

SENSIBLE nutrition is essential to health and strength. A properly balanced proportion of wholesome food is required to nourish the system. The elimination of worn-out and useless tissue continually requires new food to rebuild cell life. It is necessary that food be of the proper quality and such that it will furnish all the constituents that a healthy body needs. All food taken into the body must first be digested, but that does not finish the work, for digestion means only that the food is put into such condition that the system can assimilate it. Proper digestion prepares the food taken, and assimilation extracts the material needed to build brain, body and nerve tissue. While digestion is largely a chemical process, in which solvents both acid and alkaline are used to transform the food elements, the normal functioning of the organs which make for perfect digestion are wholly dependent upon muscular action.

In the practice of Strongfortism full consideration is given to the importance of diet. Correct eating is something about which a great many people do not know enough. They do not know how to select or how to combine different food elements, so that the greatest nourishment as well as the best money's worth may be obtained. While the principles of Strongfortism naturally cover thoroughly so important a subject as diet, there are no rules laid down that offer any difficulty in following. What is more to the point also, the personal nature of all instruction makes it possible to give to each the particular food requirements for individual needs.

Waste Matters Dangerous

STRONGFORTISM recognizes that muscular motion is necessary for the promotion and maintenance of health, as well as for the symmetrical development of the body and to correct faults of deformity. Activity is life; motion is the fundamental principle of every vital process. Muscular power and nerve force depend upon the motions of the particles that compose the body. Health demands a constant change, material must be transferred from vital organs and parts through the medium of the blood.

To maintain definite and corresponding relations so that from the food taken into the body necessary material can be used and transformed into vital energy, digestion and assimilation must be performed properly, and the resulting poisonous residue of the food thrown from the system thoroughly. The casting out of this waste matter is as necessary to health as the partaking of nourishing material. If it is not thrown off properly, a congested condition appears which clogs the system and illness results.

Cold and Catarrh

BRAIN workers and men of sedentary occupation are more subject to colds than outside active workers. Now, a cold is a very common ailment, and is the result of a congested condition of the mucous membrane, usually set up by sudden chilling, or a quick change in the temperature. The reason why brain workers more frequently contract colds is because the blood in such persons, in the majority of instances, is overloaded with impurities gathered from the system that it is constantly endeavoring to discharge through every outlet that Nature provides. Activity of the brain causes the breaking down of a large number of brain cells, and brain workers often, after excessive work, feel a stuffiness, and partial stoppage of the nasal passages because the blood in this region is surcharged with waste material.

The lack of proper activity in the lives of such workers results in a more or less sluggish condition of the circulation; consequently the blood flowing through the capillaries that gather up the waste material from the brain substance, nerve cells and muscular tissue is pretty heavily burdened. The moment a chill strikes the surface of the body, or a quick change of temperature takes place a contraction occurs which further retards the activity of the circulation. The capillaries become congested and an inflamed condition results. Repeated colds result in catarrh, which can extend through the passages of the head, throat, bronchial tubes and affects the stomach and intestines.

To eradicate catarrh it requires scientific activity of the internal muscles controlling elimination and a correction of' errors in diet, contributing to this congestion, which is constitutional in its causation. Local treatment so much advertised my relieve catarrh temporarily, but is effacement demands a thorough conditioning of the entire physical system by Strongfortism.

Constipation, the Arch Assasin

DERANGED or suppressed action of the bowels is really the basis of all departure from health and the beginning of disease. When the system becomes clogged, vital action is diminished. The most common channel that throws the system into a morbid, poisoned state, is the lower bowel or colon. When the action of this organ is impaired constipation results and particles of the poisoned refuse remaining in the bowel are constantly reabsorbed into the blood. The circulation becomes loaded with this poisonous matter; the blood vessels become weakened and distended; the circulation is retarded; the capillaries become clogged and local irritations and inflammations follow which give rise to a host of disorders.

The muscular movement of the abdominal walls and the contractile power of the tunic muscle of the large intestine bear largely upon the passing forward and expelling the waste material. The function of evacuation is almost wholly one of muscular contraction. The small intestines, which are about twenty-seven feet in length, receive the partially digested food from the stomach, and in this canal the nutritive material is separated and absorbed into the system and the residue is passed onward into the colon or large intestine. This organ is about five feet in length, and is really the receptacle for refuse material; otherwise the body would be constantly discharging. When this material remains in the lower bowel for too long a period the impurities with which it is loaded are taken up and reabsorbed by the blood, and a deranged and poisoned body results.

Physics Contrary to Nature

EVACUATION is a function of muscular contraction. When material enters into the intestines it is passed on through its entire length by the alternating contraction of muscular action, and the final expulsion is wholly muscular. It is clear, then, that to eradicate the condition of constipation, to produce healthy bowel movement, the muscles governing that function must be developed in strength and elasticity.

People tamper with Nature in their ignorance and try to do exactly the reverse. They administer purges and physics; they take pills and tablets and saline waters; all of which brings about an irritation that causes the expulsion of the fecal matter. The result is an internal convulsion of the muscles of the bowels and a further weakening. This is why so often purges arc griping, and why they cause such sharp pains that will almost double one up, which clearly shows that Nature rebels against such methods.

Oils Are Not Body Lubricants

ANOTHER idea that has been brought into vogue is that of oiling the insides. This keeping the lining of the intestines oiled up so that the contents may slide through is another instance of the ignorance of physiology that the average man possesses.

Nature has her own perfect way of providing for such demulcent secretions as may be necessary for any operation. The lining of the stomach and intestines of a healthy body are constantly making secretions such as are necessary for the purpose required of them. If they are not doing this, and trouble is experienced by the intestines becoming bound through a dry condition of these parts, it is not going to mend it by coating the parts with a filmy covering of indigestible oil to try and help the contents through.

The only way is to bring about in the diet a condition that will excite the secretions of the large intestines* at that stage, and then by a development of the muscular tone such as will enable them to function naturally and bring about evacuation as Nature intended.

This is the method in the practice of Strongfortism. It is the foundation, as it were, of the Strongfort system. It is Nature's method, and, after all, Nature's way is the only way when you are dealing with the health and welfare of your body.

Medicines will relieve constipation temporarily, but continual dosing will render the habit worse. Strongfortism without medicine will eradicate constipation completely.

I have taken up constipation because it is the most common ailment of mankind. It is responsible for many disorders and diseases. The heart, brain, kidneys, the arteries and all the organs of the body decrease in vitality; in fact, the whole system loses in resistance power and falls an easy prey to disease when constipation begins. As the practice of Strongfortism permanently removes constipation, so will it deal with the multitude of ailments and disorders with which human beings, through neglect of their body and its

How many people suffer untold miseries from Brain Fag, that tired feeling, and yet find no recuperation in their sleep. Indeed, all too often they have to endure further tortures through inability to sleep soundly, and this may develop into a kind of chronic Insomnia.

If they would but realize that one condition is but a step removed from another of equal danger, and when they begin to inter-act, it is then that complications arise which lead to disaster. Irritability is one of the simpler indications of bodily weakness. General and Nervous Debility arc well on their way when a person is unduly irritable. Indigestion, Gastritis, Biliousness, are related causes, and it depends very much on the constitution and the habits of the individual as to which ailment becomes more pronounced, although the actual cause is the same in each.

Most serious of all the complications which follow a weakened physical condition indicating Mal-nutrition, Anemia, poor Circulation as an outcome of Constipation, arc the still more treacherous ailments of an organic nature. Prostrate troubles with attendant Impotency and Sexual Debility, arc the most serious, for when the sexual force becomes weakened the whole body may be said to be at the mercy of any attack from without or within.

Strongfortism controls all such conditions, because as a Science it goes direct to fundamental causes. Such common and distressing ailments as Headache, Catarrh, Asthma, Diabetes, Torpid Liver,

Neurasthenia, Neuralgia, Lumbago, Rupture, and so forth, yield themselves speedily as the restored vitality of the body is promoted by scientific activity of the internal muscles, and sound organic functioning.

Aside from ailments due to functional derangements, of which there are still a great many not mentioned above, there are bodily defects of various troublesome sorts such as Round Shoulders, Flat Chest, Knock-Knees, Bow-legs, and so forth, which indicate conditions that may have been caused by birth, accident or neglect; but each and all of which are corrected by the application of the principles of Strongfortism.

So true to Natural Law is Strongfortism, that it may be said there is no possible ailment of the body that will not respond to the gentle, scientific practical methods of this modern science. Even so serious a condition as Rupture, may be permanently remedied, and the debilitating and degenerating influences of youthful errors, are positively overcome.

Strongfortism gives not only external muscular strength, but the more important internal strength as well; or, in other words, that vigor of the vital and functional organs which makes for untiring working efficiency and which is essential to any real health or success in life, as well as the prolongation of life and the maintenance of virility.

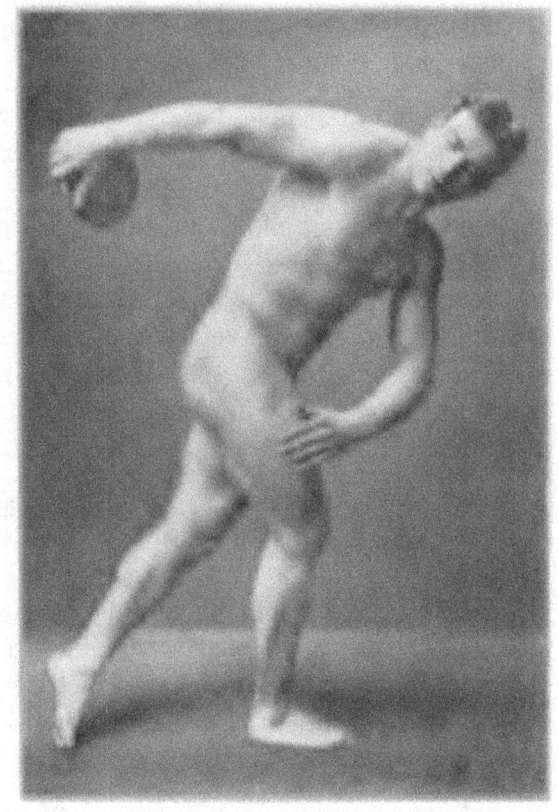

THE DISCUS THROWER
Another Famous Sculpture Piece

Drug Habits; Alcoholism

T'HE practice of Strongfortism is the most effective means to employ for subduing such habits as Alcoholism, Tobacco and Drugs. It is only the weak and lowered condition of his body that impels a man to use a stimulant or sedative. If he were strong, healthy and normal in every respect, he would have no desire for cocaine or morphine, whisky, wine or tobacco. If one is a drug fiend, chronic drinker or a victim of some other harmful habit, Strongfortism will make him strong and well and normal, give him more will power and moral courage, so that the victim once restored is always restored.

Strongfortism is a panacea for all habits that arise from physical weakness, as all bad habits do, because Strongfortism builds up Strength that resists such habits. There would be no need for Prohibition laws on liquor or any other vices if everybody practiced Strongfortism.

Youthful Errors and Devitalizing Habits

I want to say a few words to parents: If fathers and mothers would only realize the importance of having a guide and instructor covering physical fitness for their boys, one who can invite and win their confidence, I would have helpers in every home where there are growing lads. The foolish delicacy and false modesty of parents that permits children to remain in ignorance of their real nature cannot be over-estimated. It sends thousands of young men to early debility, and that is not all, for these unfortunate mistakes take out of their lives a great many of the things to which every real man looks forward with pleasure and anticipation—a wife, children and a happy family life. Thousands of young men and boys have come to me in confidence and told me of conditions that they would not confide to their parents or friends. This is natural. In conducting confidential correspondence, they can, in the privacy of their room, confide to me with frankness; needless to say, this confidence is respected. In nearly every instance they tell of the impossibility of giving their confidence to those surrounding them because of the degradation they feel that would fall upon them by so doing.

A Word to Parents

PARENTS ought to have their sons take up the practice of Strongfortism to develop that manliness, that courage, that moral fibre and strength of purpose that would lead them onward and upward and prevent the very existence of degenerative influences. The realization of the effects of pernicious habits and its results on posterity has made eugenics one of the most vital subjects of the day, and it is safe to say the time is not distant when marriage under these circumstances will be a crime. A casual observation of the statistics of idiots, degenerates, deformed children, show beyond dispute a few of the terrible results of such deplorable habits and the asylums are filled with victims who have become enslaved, and, in most cases, through no fault of their own.

Any youth or young man who has had the misfortune to thus endanger his career should take immediate steps toward its eradication. Continuance will sap the vitality to the utmost and undermine the constitution. It will surely lead to other and even more serious ills if neglected for any length of time. It is my belief that no one is bad because he wants to be, but simply because he is powerless to free himself from the cause of his downfall, but to delay in taking progressive steps to overcome such condition only paves the way to physical deterioration and to mental perversion and moral degradation. So such a matter demands Immediate Attention, and the sooner it is attended to the better for the sufferer. I appeal to every young man addicted to such habit, I invite his confidence, assuring him of my personal sympathy and help, as my special methods and advice have never failed to entirely remedy all cases of this kind and restore to normal health.

Premature Decay; Loss of Sexual Power

WHEN excesses have been continued until the virile powers have been impaired and manhood begins to sway in the balance, it is useless to turn to stimulants, medicines or other artificial means to regain permanent strength and restoration. The much heralded gland treatment is an illustration of the extent and seriousness of this physical condition. Prof. Steinach, of Vienna, an authority on the subject decries the commercializing of what so far has been merely scientific investigation. Tablets cannot possibly have any restorative effects in rebuilding glands. The effects of such are not restorative, and results are not lasting; on the contrary, use of drugs and tonics will, in a short time, still lower the virile forces to a greater degree, for, the stimulation being temporary, the resulting reflex occurring brings greater degeneracy until restoration becomes impossible. Neither does electricity reach the seat of the trouble.

The diminished power and apparently total loss of power indicates that the nerve centers have become morbid and unhealthy, and that there is a faulty functional condition of the spinal cord. In other words, the nerve system has degenerated in consequence of being depleted of material, without being replenished and supplied by a healthy deposit from a rich and nourishment-laden blood. The glands also cannot store secretions because of the lack of elements in the system that furnish the source of supply.

Strongfortism will effect a radical and constitutional change. There is a positive regain of body tone and vigor of mind; the sexual weakness disappears and there is a complete restoration of general health and sexual functions. The results are remarkable in many instances, often surprising pupil and friend by the improvement in looks and rejuvenated appearance.

Impotency May Be Overcome

VERY frequently loss of manhood presents itself by certain symptoms that point to its commencement, premature ejection, continual losses, unconscious ciriissions, diminishment in size of organs of generation, slow and short response; all indicate impairment and progress toward impotency. Often this condition becomes apparent at an early age, even before the summit of vigor and strength ought to have been reached.

There is nothing beyond marvel in the results produced by Strongfortism; there is no creating anew; Nature is wholesomely assisted in restoring the balance and m rebuilding and repairing. The results appear marvelous, just as though some creative process was brought into play. Strongfortism has proven that man can regain his virility and retain vigor and power until advanced age. Wide and valuable experience enables the assurance to be given to every man threatened with premature decay that they can be fully restored through Strongfortism.

Prostate Troubles

THE Prostate Gland is a vitally important member of the reproductive organs. It is a muscular structure and being the center of that great network of nerves known as the "Sexual Plexus," any unnatural condition that affects it seriously undermines the health, strength and vitality. It contains so many important nerves and is so intimately associated with the Spinal Cord and the Brain that it is often called "Man's Second Brain." Disorders of this gland, whether arising from Masturbation, Excesses, Venereal Infection, Constipation or any other condition that impairs the purity and efficiency of the blood, immediately affects every part of the Body and Brain. It is a most common cause of urinary troubles, sexual weakness, impotency and lost power, and often affects the mental faculties, bringing about Poor Memory, Morbidness, Super-Sensitiveness, Irritability, Self-Consciousness, Lack of Concentration, Melancholia, Fear, etc. Drugs, massage,, electricity and all such applications fail to permanently benefit the weakened or diseased Prostrate Gland because this important organ can only be restored to normal health through purifying the blood, rehabilitating the nerves, and building up the general resistance and vitality. The Science of Strongfortism contains all that is effective, safe and sensible to aid Nature in overcoming inflammation and enlargement of the Prostrate Gland and in restoring it and all other parts of the Body and Brain to normal health and efficiency.

Strongfortism and Complications

MANY pupils upon enrollment present complications of disorders; that is, there is frequently a constipated condition and with this hemorrhoids and rupture, or perhaps, in some other instance, there would be stomach disorders, indigestion, dyspepsia, constipation and heart trouble. It is readily seen, therefore, that the course of Strongfortism must be arranged to suit the need of such sufferers to overcome the ailments and disorders, and also to specifically strengthen the muscular tissues. In the first instance deterioration and weakness of the abdominal muscles permitted the rupture, and in the other instance the movements of the exercises must be so modified that functional activity to the organs is established without bringing an undue strain to the heart, until it is restored to normal function. Instructions and guidance are always therefore given, and the practice of the course arranged to suit the need of each individual pupil, whether complications exist or not. The practice of Strongfortism as instructed takes into consideration the individual tendency of the pupil enrolled, as well as the conditions presented.

One great advantage of the system of Strongfortism is the fact that it positively accomplishes a symmetrical development of the entire body. The method of bringing this about is that of developing each muscle separately by the use of special individual exercises for each and every part of the body, no muscle or group of muscles being overlooked. Defective or weakened parts arc given special attention so that the body will become uniformly strong throughout.

The movements of the body as directed to meet the requirements of the individuals are of great value without apparatus of any kind, but in order to obtain the very best results and to secure the desired resistance, many of these movements are performed witli the aid of resistance-increasing dumb-bells that can be made to vary in weight approximately from four to ten pounds, the variation depending upon the strength and condition of the pupil practicing. Upon careful consideration of the condition of each pupil, it is determined just at what weight the dumb-bell should be used when beginning the course.

The dumb-bell furnishes the best form of apparatus and the most satisfactory method of resistance in increasing physical development that can be used. Better results can be accomplished with them in the particular exercises than through any other means.

Are You Too Fat?

IF you are burdened with superfluous flesh you can lose your burden. Obesity has its causes, like everything else, and these causes arc found chiefly in the lack of physical activity and in dietetic errors. There is no such thing as man being unable to reduce his weight, no matter what his belief about it being "constitutional" or "temperamental" in his case. If only he will adopt proper measures, he can reduce flesh until he is down to a normal, natural weight, a point at which his health and efficiency will be the very' greatest possible for him.

The Strongfort reducing system is easily applied and strikes directly at the parts that harbor the superfluous flesh, removing it in a short time. Common-sense and simple suggestions about clothing and food are given. The wearing of tight garments and things of that kind to hide the excessive fat arc positively dangerous, and instead of hiding the trouble, such methods show it up more. Strongfortism does not lower the vitality in the slightest, as these wrong methods do. On the contrary, every part will be strengthened and restored to its proper form in an easy, pleasant and natural manner.

Too much stress cannot be laid upon the dangers of chemical fat reducers, put out in the form o-f lotions, crcalns, etc. Drugs are of as little value for external application as for internal. There have been some disastrous results following such methods, and some law suits have been the outcome, where bodily injury has followed the use of such applications

Are You Too Skinny?

EMACIATION in many cases is due to digestive difficulties or failings, but perhaps more frequently to the lack of general bodily vigor and functional tone which follow persistent neglect of exercise, coupled with a conspicuous lack of muscular development. The individual is all "run down." Scientific natural methods are wanted, instead of tablets and "tonics." If your food doesn't nourish you, your body is STARVED, no matter how much and what you cat. In thin persons a great deal of the food elements that should go toward building flesh, muscle and tissue passes off without having fulfilled the purpose for which it was intended. Functional activity must be restored by a thorough systematic building up or organic strength, so that the organs whose duty it is to do so can separate the food, retaining the good for the building up of health and strength and allowing the waste to be carried away naturally. "Flesh- producers," so-called, like iron-compounds, etc., like fat reducers, should be abstained from. The only safe and sane way to gain or lose weight is by close adherence to Natural Law, for Nature always has a tendency to equalize and normalize everything over which she has any influence, and if one lives and acts according to Natural law, the results will be the making in a perfectly natural way, of a normal, well proportioned body. In addition to giving you scientific exercises to promote assimilative vigor, special instructions are given in regard to diet which will tell you just what elements of food contain the materials necessary. This means that you will know which of the staple articles of food are best suited to your individual requirements, and therefore sure to produce the results you want. Special instructions and expert advice cover not only external, but also internal muscles and organs; thus assimilative vigor is assured as well as correct muscular development.

Whether too fat or too thin, Strongfortism will bring you back to the normal, to your best weight and the best of health.

Increasing Your Height

A NY specific increase in height by irksome and unnatural methods, such as pulling, forcing, stretching, etc., will only harm; increased height cannot come from that sort of thing. To increase your height, you require a thoroughly sound development of your whole body so that your height may increase proportionately. Many people, even though not humped or round-shouldered, are still not as tall as they might be, and I believe anyone will increase his height by adopting my methods, as by them the spine will be thoroughly straightened, all the muscles of the back will be fully developed and strengthened and the cartilages extended to the greatest natural limit. At any rate you will grow as tall as Nature will permit, without interfering with its proper functions. Numbers of pupils have thus increased their height.

Internal Muscular Development

WHEN the muscles are not developed the body becomes diseased, weak, and falls into decay. A weakness or relaxation of the muscles of the back allows the body to drop into unsightly and unhealthy positions. The ribs fall inward, compressing the lungs, decreasing the lung capacity and preventing normal breathing and the necessary purification of the blood. It also limits the action of the heart by limiting the space for its expansion. It forces all the vitality important internal organs downward. It thus lowers the vigor and free functioning of the system. You must not expect the internal muscles to be in a better condition than the external ones. As a matter of fact, the internal muscles arc often much weaker than the external. These conditions can be quickly corrected by my scientifically arranged exercises. The effect upon the activities of the internal organs is most remarkable, quickly starting the harmonious flow of the life forces and inducing normal functioning of the vital organs.

Pleasant, Safe and Profitable

WHEN you think of improving your health and strength, you should be careful to have the best advice. You want personal help to suit your condition, not a mere set of exercises, one and all alike, such as some self-styled Physical directors send out in connection with a rubber or spring stretching exerciser. It is on the exercisers they sell they expect to make their profit.

I have been teaching for over 25 years and I know how. It will not be physical torture or too much like work. You will find pleasure all the way through, as the methods are agreeably interesting.

Bodily Movements Photographed

A feature of the Strongfort Course is that the bodily movements are shown by means of photographs, and not by little drawings. I posed for these photographs myself, showing in detail and with the greatest accuracy just how each movement should be made. It enables a pupil to see very clearly the exact movements to be made for his ailment or condition.

What Strongfortism Gives

YOUR Course in Strongfortism is all individual and personal. Your needs are carefully studied and your age, height, weight, lack of development, as well as the condition of your stomach, bowels and vital organs, the circulation, nervous system and any diseases or weaknesses that may be present, are particularly taken into

Your lessons arc prepared accordingly, with all needed instruction as to your mode of living, diet, specially arranged exercises, baths and helpful directions to meet your requirements, including your sexual life. Your progress during the entire time is carefully watched. You are guided and directed and given every assistance. The confidential nature of the lessons make it impossible for you to go wrong.

For All Ages and Condition

I prepare courses for all conditions—for men and women, for children and for the aged, for the invalid in bed, for the tot whose development is fault}', for the active business man and for the laboring man. I meet the requirements of the society woman, who must have a fresh, velvety complexion, firm, healthy flesh with beauty of form and grace of movement. I fill the needs of the aged, whose tottering footsteps I make firm, filling their forms with the fire of returning health and vigor.

The weakling is developed and inspired with the mastery of mental power and physical perfection—the glorious crown of MANHOOD. The dyspeptic and neurotic, whose system is wracked by disease, finds rebirth in the quickening pulse of a revitalized body, vibrant with health and energy.

Charges Are Moderate

IN order to reach all in need of my services I make my charges the lowest consistent with efficient service. Efficiency has been the key of my success. You can get books and pamphlets giving so-called "Physical Culture" exercises. There are also self-styled professors and teachers selling courses. I warn you against these things. The cheap, prepared, stereotyped course, arranged by an inexperienced, incompetent person will do no good and likely much harm.

My charges arc modest whether you want a Course to develop your muscles and improve the symmetry of your form, or overcome some dread weakness or disease.

STRONGFORTISM is the key which unlocks Nature's storehouse of vital energy. It reaches and develops the inner muscles which control the vital organs, generating the Life Forces. Enroll today and start on that road which leads to Physical Health, Strength and Vitality Supreme, and you will realize the joys of the ABUNDANT LIFE.

Address all letters to LIONEL STRONGFORT, The Strongfort Institute, Newark, New Jersey, U. S. A.